AROMATHERAPY – THE BABY BOOK

by Marion Del Gaudio Mak

Published by
Amberwood Publishing Ltd
Park Corner, Park Horsley, East Horsley, Surrey KT24 5RZ
Tel: 01483 570821 Fax: 01483 282321

PLANTLIFE

The Natural History Museum, Cromwell Road, London SW7 5BD

Registered Charity No. 328576

Amberwood Publishing supports the Plantlife Charity,
Britain's only charity exclusively dedicated to saving wild plants.

ISBN 1-899308-18-0

Cover design by Howland Northover
Photography by Mark Mak

Printed in Great Britain

CONTENTS

About the Author

Marion Del Gaudio Mak is a beauty therapist and aromatherapist currently lecturing at Southport College of Art and Technology. She is programme manager for beauty therapy, aromatherapy and sports therapy and is responsible for a range of courses incorporating, holistic therapy, reflexology, shiatsu, indian head massage and baby massage.

Marion has been an external examiner for the *International Health and Beauty Council* and is now an external assessor and verifier for them. She is also a member of *The Federation of Holistic Therapists* and *The International Federation of Aromatherapists*.

As a freelance consultant and trainer for beauty therapy and hairdressing salons her work often takes her overseas. She is regularly invited to speak to groups on the subject of aromatherapy.

Acknowledgements

I would like to thank Mum and Papa for supporting me through my years at college, Concetta and Luigi for trying my recipes, Mark for technical assistance and unlimited patience and Sophie, for being my youngest guinea pig and aromatherapy fan. I would also like to thank all my special friends, colleagues, and students and who have had so much faith in me.

Thanks also to June Crisp of Amberwood Publishing Limited.

Note to Reader

Whilst the author has made every effort to ensure that the contents of this book are accurate in every particular, it is not intended to be regarded as a substitute for professional medical advice under treatment. The reader is urged to give careful consideration to any difficulties which he or she is experiencing with their own health and to consult their General Practitioner if uncertain as to its cause or nature. Neither the author nor the publisher can accept any legal responsibility for any health problem which results from use of the self-help methods described.

Foreword

As an experienced and qualified beauty therapist, aroma-therapist and holistic therapist, currently lecturing in these subjects, I feel that everyone should be aware of the benefits of aromatherapy and massage. I believe in natural and holistic methods for the treatment and prevention of ailments and that good health comes from combining a natural and wholesome diet with exercise and sufficient sleep. A healthy lifestyle should be something the whole family can enjoy and this should commence from birth.

The benefits of massage on the newborn infant have been proven to be effective for many centuries. This guide to massage for the infant or child is straightforward and easy to follow, it is suitable for the new mother and her baby and can be of use for children up to the age of ten. It also gives information on the effects and uses of essential oils for massage and the treatment of minor ailments. The recipes given are those which I have formulated from experience and are simple and effective to use.

Massage can be tried at home on healthy infants and children, however, if medical conditions are present or there are complications, I would recommend seeking advice from a medical professional.

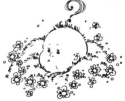

1 Introduction to baby massage

Massage is the manipulation of the soft tissues of the body, but in reality it is so much more. It is touch, comfort, reassurance, nurturing, pleasure, relaxation, pain relief, and communication.

Massage has so many valuable and lasting effects, for example increasing blood and lymphatic flow bringing nutrients to the tissues and replenishing vital elements to all the body systems. The nervous system is affected in a positive manner by massage and in general, an overall sense of well being will result.

The effects of massage on babies and children has for centuries been noted by many communities around the world.

As an essential part of daily routine, mothers would massage their babies soon after birth to increase the maternal bond and develop their relationship with their new offspring.

Massage would keep skin soft and protected and ensure that muscles and joints were healthy and supple.

During these daily massage sessions mother and baby formed a special language which helped them to get to know each other and to establish vital contact which is so important for the well being of the infant.

These precious moments often allowed the mother to identify at an early stage, any potential signs of skin or health problems and wherever possible, deal with them.

These simple and ancient techniques of early infant care were a natural and important part of life however, in today's modern society, touch is often discouraged and physical contact kept to a minimum.

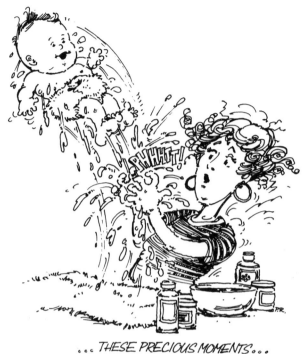

... *THESE PRECIOUS MOMENTS* ...

Today, there are many labour saving methods of infant care that have led perhaps to the more natural and traditional methods of child care being forgotten. This has created a society which has favoured little physical contact and therefore many communities have lost the special and caring techniques which incorporate parental massage.

Fortunately, there is a rise in the popularity of natural health remedies, herbal medicines and aromatherapy as more people are developing an awareness of personal health and the importance of prevention and not cure! It makes sense therefore that if natural preparations are being chosen to treat or prevent ailments, other ancient traditions are again being utilised.

2 | Infant care around the world

Many different communities around the world have special rituals of infant care that incorporate some form of baby massage. Chinese, Indian, Lebanese, Arab, Russian, Italian and French families all report that they had particular methods of

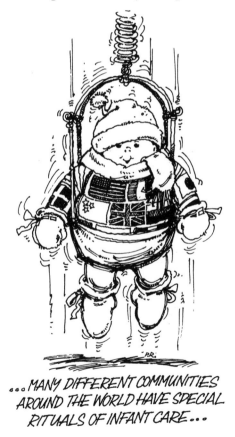

...MANY DIFFERENT COMMUNITIES AROUND THE WORLD HAVE SPECIAL RITUALS OF INFANT CARE...

infant care which were carried out by either the mother, the grandmother or extended family members and consisted of one or several of the following: massage, binding, wrapping, cocooning, swaddling, anointing, bathing, caressing. Massage would take place soon after the birth of the baby and continue daily for several years. The routine would obviously vary but whether it simply be the stroking of the infants brow or the most complex massage routine, the outcome would invariably be the same, ie to soothe and calm and impart a sense of well being, whilst developing and strengthening the maternal or paternal bond between parent and child.

Binding or wrapping infants serves to cocoon and surround them securely, keeping them warm and imparting a sense of security and comfort.

Bathing the infant, often before massage and with specially prepared herbal concoctions or essential oils, ensures that the relaxation process is enhanced.

3 | Preparing for massage

It is important that the 'time is right' before commencing massage so that maximum benefits may be obtained by both the child and the mother or the massage giver. The massage giver could be either parent or member of the family with the parents permission. Often the father feels that being involved in this way gives him a purpose when the new baby comes into the family and requires so much maternal care, ie breast feeding, and often fathers tend to feel left out! Older sisters or brothers can also be included and again, this allows them to feel that they have an important role to play within the family. The participation of all family members helps to dispel any jealousy that may occur when the new baby arrives if together the family establish a routine and spend time together. Ensure that the infant or child is comfortable with the idea of the massage and encourage them to feel that this is their special time!

Let the infant or child have a special teddy or toy and use a warm fluffy towel as a wrap or to lie on. Use the same items for each massage session in order that the infant becomes familiar with these items and therefore learns to associate them with the pleasures of massage.

Choose a warm, peaceful environment free from interruptions and stresses. Soft music may help to create a pleasant atmosphere. An essential oil diffuser to fragrance the room is a good way to enhance relaxation, however exercise caution in the choice of essential oil. Mandarin is an excellent choice for infants and children with its gentle, soothing properties.

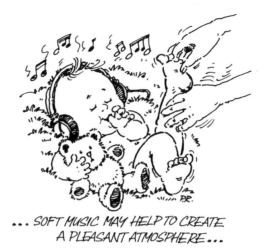

... *SOFT MUSIC MAY HELP TO CREATE*
A PLEASANT ATMOSPHERE ...

Make sure that you are wearing loose comfortable clothing which will allow you to kneel on the floor and bend with ease. Your nails should be short, free from enamel and scrupulously clean. No jewellery should be worn to prevent scratching and damaging delicate skin tissue.

Choose a suitable massage medium from those listed in this book, as an approximate guide 10mls should be sufficient although more or less may be required according to the size of the infant or child or the dryness of the skin. It may however, be wise to practice the massage routine without oil until you become proficient.

Bathe the infant and gently pat the skin dry. Place the infant onto the warm towel which is laid out on the floor.

Look into the infants eyes and ensure that you maintain constant eye contact. This is a good form of communication and can help to build a strong bond between infant and massage giver. Make the initial contact with the infant gentle but firm and very positive. This is important to ensure that the infant can sense that you mean no harm and that you can instill confidence which will allow the infant to relax and enjoy the massage.

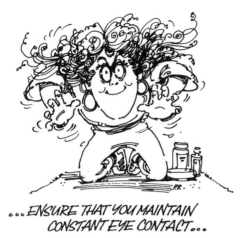

... ENSURE THAT YOU MAINTAIN CONSTANT EYE CONTACT ...

Begin by gently but firmly taking hold of the infants hands and pressing for a moment. Talk to the infant in quiet tones whilst maintaining eye contact. When you are sure that you have gained the confidence of the infant, you .should commence the massage routine.

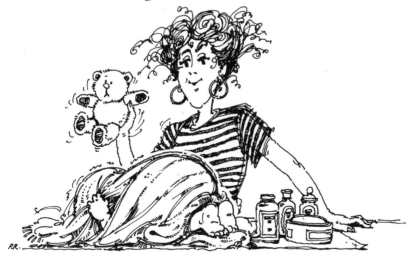

... THERE ARE CERTAIN CONDITIONS WHERE MASSAGE SHOULD NOT BE GIVEN ...

Remember, that if the infant appears to be upset, distressed or unhappy in anyway, the massage should stop immediately.

When not to massage

There are certain conditions where massage should not be given and if these conditions are present, or if you are simply unsure, it is advisable to seek advice from a qualified aromatherapist. It is always wise to be cautious.

Contra indications

Serious medical conditions
Medication
Recent surgery
Broken bones
Open wounds
Infections – fungal, viral, bacterial
Allergies (avoid nut carrier oils)
Colds and influenza
General debility
Fever
Immediately after feeding
Infant hungry
Infant tired, restless, irritated

4 | The massage giver

The massage giver must expect to give time, patience, care and affection to the infant, and should be sensitive to the infant's moods and the needs of the infant at each massage session.

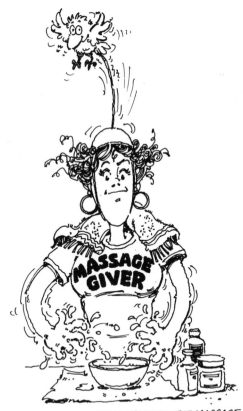

...IT IS IMPORTANT THAT BEFORE THE MASSAGE BEGINS THE RIGHT ATMOSPHERE IS CREATED...

The massage giver should intuitively know when to massage and when to stop. The infant is vulnerable and helpless and will ultimately put its trust in the hands of the massage giver.

It should be remembered that the gift of massage is valuable and can be a useful therapy which can enable the massage giver and the child to develop a special bond as a result of a transfer of positive energy.

It is important that before the massage begins the right atmosphere is created and the mood or attitude of the child is assessed as calm and responsive.

5 | Simple massage techniques

Massage techniques are best kept as simple as possible and the movements listed below are formulated to make an easy to follow routine.

When you have practiced and become proficient at massage, you may be able to devise your own gentle movements and create a personalised routine to suite the individual baby or child.

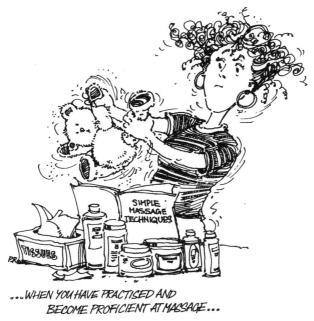

...WHEN YOU HAVE PRACTISED AND
BECOME PROFICIENT AT MASSAGE...

Always use an even pressure for all the massage strokes and start with strokes and movements towards the heart, this will help the blood flow. Repeat each movement at least three times on the chosen area. Always complete the routine on one part of the body before beginning on the next.

Bear in mind that the movements may have to be modified slightly according to the size of the area you are working on and that sometimes movements will have to be performed with finger or thumb if there is simply no space to work with all fingers or the palm of the hand.

Begin the massage by massaging the arms, legs, chest, abdomen, face and then finally the back.

Stroking – is literally a 'stroking' action which is performed by sliding fingers or hand upwards or outwards on the area being treated. This movement may be performed with light or firm pressure.

Milking – is a movement which is performed in a similar method to 'milking' a cow. The fingers encircle the limb and firmly pull downwards working up the limb with alternate hands.

Four finger stroking – is exactly the same as *stroking* but performed solely with the fingertips. A gentle movement to stimulate the nerve endings.

Squeezing – is a firm squeezing action performed in a rhythmic manner with the thumbs and fingers supporting the area and the palm giving extra pressure. This movement is performed upwards.

Bending and flexing – is a passive movement performed on the joints by bending and then flexing the arms and legs to strengthen and give flexibility.

Massaging the sides – is a movement performed on the sides of the body and the sides of the face. The movement is performed with all the fingers in circular movements.

Kneading – is a squeezing action similar to that of 'kneading' dough performed firmly over the area with fingertips and palm.

Wringing – is a grasping and squeezing action performed with one hand initially moving the flesh towards the second hand and gently twisting. This may be also performed with the fingers on smaller areas.

Thumb circling – is a circling action performed with the thumbs working systematically over the area.

6 | The massage routine

The arms
Work from fingertips right up to the shoulder.

1. Stroking
2. Thumb circling
3. Squeezing
4. Milking
5. Bend and flex
6. Stroking

The legs
Work from the toes right up to the thigh.

1. Stroking
2. Thumb circling
3. Squeezing
4. Milking
5. Bend and flex
6. Stroking

The neck and chest
Work from the neck, over shoulders and down over chest.

1. Stroking
2. Finger circling
3. Thumb circling
4. Four finger stroking
5. Stroking

The abdomen
Work from the lower abdomen upwards to the sternum.

1. Stroking
2. Finger circling
3. Kneading
4. Wringing
5. Four finger stroking
6. Stroking

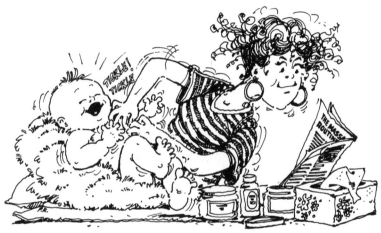

...WORK FROM THE LOWER ABDOMEN UPWARDS TO THE STERNUM...

The back
Work from the buttocks upwards to shoulders.

1. Stroking
2. Finger circling
3. Kneading
4. Wringing
5. Four finger stroking
6. Stroking

7 | Essential oils and baby massage

Essential oils are powerful, volatile natural essences which are obtained from plants and flowers. Essential oils are used successfully in the treatment of a variety of conditions. Have caution when using essential oils on or near to babies and small children. Essential oils must not be taken internally.

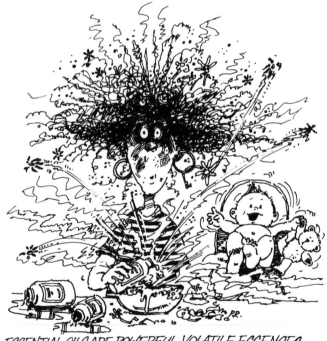

...ESSENTIAL OILS ARE POWERFUL, VOLATILE ESSENCES WHICH ARE OBTAINED FROM PLANTS AND FLOWERS...
...ALWAYS USE EXTREME CAUTION...

For small children, blending proportions must not exceed 1% and babies require even smaller dosage, no more than ½% and even less if in doubt, ie 1 to 2 parts essential oil to 100 parts carrier oil. Never be tempted to increase dosage as essential oils are potent. ALWAYS USE EXTREME CAUTION AND IF UNSURE CONSULT A PROFESSIONAL AROMATHERAPIST.

Examples of proportions for blending

Carrier Oil

200 drops of carrier oil = 10ml carrier oil
400 drops of carrier oil = 20ml carrier oil
1000 drops of carrier oil = 50ml carrier oil

Essential Oil

To 10ml carrier oil maximum drops of essential oil = 1-2
To 20ml carrier oil maximum drops of essential oil = 4
To 50ml carrier oil maximum drops of essential oil = 6
(depending on the size of the infant or child)

8 | Synergistic blending

When a recipe calls for more than one essential oil and you want to keep the blending proportions to a minimum it is useful to prepare a synergistic blend.

Preparing a synergistic blend

Add 1 drop of each essential oil into an amber glass bottle then gently mix. You may now add the required number of drops, ie 1 to the chosen carrier medium. Save the remaining drops for future use. This method strengthens the properties of the oils and still allows minimal amounts of essential oils to be added to the carrier.

9 | Safety precautions and hazards

Essential oils must be treated with great respect as they are potent chemical substances and can be dangerous if not used correctly. Essential oils may be hazardous to the body and may result in reactions in certain individuals. Essential oils must not be taken internally or applied to the eyes or delicate mucous membranes. In order to check whether a sensitivity or allergic reaction will occur with essential oils, it is important to carry out a skin sensitivity test prior to using the chosen blend of essential oils.

A skin sensitivity test should be carried out twenty-four hours prior to using essential oils. It must also be remembered that an allergy may develop at any time regardless of prior history and in the case of infants, extra caution must be taken.

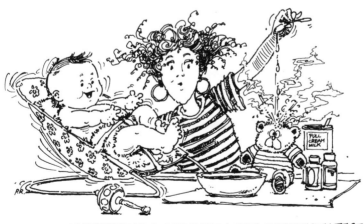

... IT IS IMPORTANT TO CARRY OUT A SKIN SENSITIVITY TEST PRIOR TO USING THE CHOSEN BLEND OF ESSENTIAL OILS...

If an essential oil is accidentally spilt onto the skin, the area should be flooded with a vegetable carrier oil which will dilute the effects of the essential oil. If essential oils accidentally enter the eyes flush copiously with distilled or sterile water. Always seek medical help if you are unsure. Neat essential oils must not be applied to the skin as they are too concentrated and will damage skin tissue. Essential oils should be mixed in a vegetable carrier oil when used topically. Mineral oils and alcohol are not regarded as suitable carrier media for aromatherapy use. Water may be added when making up a compress and for baths and must be agitated well in order to disperse the droplets of essential oil thoroughly. To ensure adequate dispersal of essential oils in the bath add them to a tablespoon of full cream milk before putting into the water.

Extra care must be taken when using essential oils in diffusers around infants and children as they may experience strong reactions to certain essential oils.

Prior to the use of essential oils for baby massage, the following instructions should apply:

Skin sensitivity test

1. Blend required essential oils with carrier oil.
2. Wash and dry a small area of skin on the inner elbow.
3. Using a cotton bud, apply essential oil blend to the area.
4. Cover the area with plaster and leave for 24–48 hours.
5. If irritation occurs, remove plaster and flood area with neat carrier oil.
6. If no adverse reactions are displayed, treatment may commence.

If a reaction has developed this procedure must be repeated with other blends until a suitable combination is reached.

Remember that a careful check should be kept on the test area to ensure that the infant does not suffer any discomfort from this test.

10 | Suitable essential oils for babies and children

Although there are many essential oils available, it is wise to choose from only a few gentle oils which will be suitable for babies and children and the conditions which often require treatment in the early years. Bear in mind that essential oils are potent natural essences and some oils may be extremely hazardous to the small infant if used indiscriminately.

The essential oils listed below have been chosen for their gentle but powerful properties and their usefulness in treating a wide variety of conditions successfully.

CHAMOMILE ROMAN *Anthemis nobilis*
PROPERTIES – Antiseptic, antibacterial, antispasmodic, digestive, sedative, tonic.
USES – Bathing, skin care, nappy rashes, eczema, colic, earache, teething, restlessness.

EUCALYPTUS *Eucalyptus globulus*
PROPERTIES – Antiseptic, analgesic, antiviral, decongestant, expectorant.
USES – Colds, flu, congestion, coughs, sinus.

FENNEL (SWEET) *Foeniculum vulgare*
PROPERTIES – Anti-inflammatory, antiseptic, antispasmodic, digestive, tonic.
USES – Colic, hiccough, asthma, constipation, nausea, digestive problems.

LAVENDER *Lavendula officianalis*
PROPERTIES – Antiseptic, antibacterial, antitoxic, anti-spasmodic, sedative.
USES – Bathing, skincare, massage, relaxation, colds, infections.

MANDARIN *Citrus reticulata*
PROPERTIES – Antiseptic, antispasmodic, digestive, laxative, sedative, tonic.
USES – Skincare, bathing, insomnia, hiccoughs, indigestion, constipation, relaxation.

NEROLI *Citrus aurantium*
PROPERTIES – Antiseptic, antispasmodic, antibacterial, digestive, fungicidal, tonic.
USES – Skincare, bathing, colic, massage, indigestion, stress, relaxation.

PEPPERMINT *Mentha piperita*
PROPERTIES – Analgesic, digestive, antiseptic, decongestant.
USES – Headaches, colic, congestion, digestive problems.

ROSE (DAMASCENA) *Rosa damascena*
PROPERTIES – Antiseptic, antitoxic, sedative.
USES – Bathing, skincare, restlessness, bed wetting.

TEA TREE *Melaleuca alternifolia*
PROPERTIES – Antiseptic, antibacterial, anti-inflammatory, antiviral, fungicidal, expectorant.
USES – Bathing, skincare, nappy rashes, asthma, colds, coughs, sinusitis, thrush, infections.

11 | Carrier oils

Carrier oils are non-volatile substances which are extracted from the seeds of fruits, flowers and nuts. Carrier oils are used as a medium for essential oil application. A carrier oil should be chosen for its specific properties in relation to the type of skin or area of the body to which it will be applied. Some carrier oils have a distinct colour or odour and this should be taken into account when choosing in order to avoid heavy odours and staining of linen and clothing. Always purchase carrier oils in small amounts to ensure freshness, taking care that they are 'Cold Pressed', which means that they have been obtained from natural sources.

The pure, natural and unrefined carrier oils should be obtained from a reputable supplier who should be able to confirm the process by which the oil was obtained. Cold pressed carrier oils may turn slightly cloudy when stored at low temperatures, and as previously explained, may possess a strong odour.

Carrier oils should always be stored in amber glass bottles with airtight lids as they may turn rancid if exposed to the air. Wheatgerm is the exception to this and is an excellent natural antioxidant. Wheatgerm may be added at 5% to all blends to prolong shelf life.

A note of caution when choosing carrier oils, check that the infant is not sensitive, or allergic to any of the substances ie, the natural fruits, flowers or nuts from which the carrier oils are derived. It is wise to avoid nut oils, especially peanut oils on newborn infants and small children prone to sensitivity to avoid the possibility of sensitisation. Choose instead carriers which are derived from fruits, flowers or other natural sources. The exception to this rule appears to be sweet almond oil which has gentle, soothing properties suitable for delicate skin.

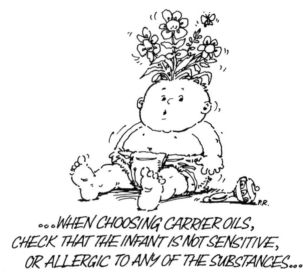

∘∘∘*WHEN CHOOSING CARRIER OILS,*
CHECK THAT THE INFANT IS NOT SENSITIVE,
OR ALLERGIC TO ANY OF THE SUBSTANCES∘∘∘

Some carrier oils are rather expensive and may be used as a percentage of the total carrier blend with another carrier oil, however, if cost is not a consideration these carrier oils may be used as 100% blend. Take into account the viscosity and texture of the oil and also the texture and condition of the infant's skin when choosing a carrier oil.

APRICOT KERNEL OIL – Pale gold in colour. Useful for sensitive, inflammed and dry skin. May be used as 100% dilution.

AVOCADO PEAR OIL – Dark green in colour. Excellent for dry, dehydrated skin and eczema. Use as a 10% dilution.

BORAGE SEED OIL – Pale yellow in colour. Suitable for psoriasis and dry skin. Use as a 10% dilution.

CORN OIL – Pale yellow in colour. Soothing for all skin types. May be used as 100% dilution.

EVENING PRIMROSE OIL – Pale yellow in colour, rich in gamma linolenic acid. Recommended for eczema, psoriasis, dry and delicate skin. Use as a 10% dilution.

GRAPESEED OIL – Almost colourless, may be used for all skin types. Makes a good, light textured carrier oil. May be used as 100% dilution.

JOJOBA – Pale golden, a liquid wax which mimics natural collagen. Excellent for all skin types especially oily and sensitive. Good for haircare and the scalp. May be used as 100% dilution.

OLIVE OIL – Green in colour. Excellent for skincare. May be used as 100% dilution.

PASSION FLOWER OIL – Golden in colour, a fine textured oil, useful for delicate skin. May be used as a 10% dilution.

ROSE HIP OIL – Almost colourless. Excellent for skincare, particularly delicate, dry skins. May be used as a 10% dilution.

SAFFLOWER OIL – Pale yellow in colour. Excellent for skincare, may be used for all skin types. May be used as a 10% dilution.

SESAME OIL – Dark golden in colour, excellent for the body. May be used as a 10% dilution.

SOYA BEAN OIL – Pale yellow in colour, a good massage base, useful for all skin types. May be used as 100% dilution.

SUNFLOWER OIL – Pale yellow in colour. Useful for all skin types. May be used as 100% dilution.

SWEET ALMOND OIL – Golden in colour. Excellent for dry, delicate skin, inflammation and itching. May be used as a 100% dilution.

WHEATGERM OIL – Deep orange in colour. Suitable for eczema, psoriasis and dry skin. Use as a 10% dilution.

12 | Methods of using essential oils for infant care

There are many ways essential oils may be used every day to impart a sense of well being and balance. Using essential oils need not be a time consuming process. Aromatherapy is so simple and effective it can be incorporated into the daily routine of the infant or child and utilised whenever required. Do not exceed the recommended dosage when using essential oils, however, you may decrease the dosage if required.

Air fresheners – Fill a plant spray with warm water. Add essential oils and spray into the air to kill bacteria and fragrance the environment. Avoid polished surfaces. Useful for environmental hygiene and mood enhancing.

Compress – Dip a pad of linen or cotton wool into a basin of water in which a drop of essential oil has been added. Apply to the affected area. Hot or cold water may be used according to the condition being treated. Useful for irritations, rashes, fevers, bites or boils.

Direct application – Lavender and Tea Tree are the only essential oils which may safely be applied directly to the skin, however it is not recommended that neat essential oils are used on very small infants and should be used with caution on all children. Useful for cuts, burns, bruises, boils, bites, spots etc.

Footbath – Add 1 drop of essential oil to a footbath using the same method as for baths. Useful for chaffed skin, blisters, tired feet, verrucas and minor infections.

Baths – Add drops of essential oils to the bathing water. Use up to 2 drops of essential oil mixed into a tablespoon of full cream milk and agitate the water to aid dispersal of essential oils. For maximum benefit the infant should remain in the water to allow the essential oils to work. Alternatively, add essential oils to the carrier oil of your choice, massage the skin before entering the bath. Always ensure that the temperature of the water is not too high and choose lukewarm to warm water to avoid discomfort. Baths are useful for general hygiene or to treat specific conditions.

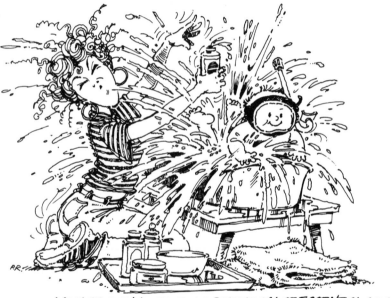

... AGITATE THE WATER TO AID DISPERSAL OF ESSENTIAL OILS...

Hygiene in the home – As essential oils are powerful antiseptic and antibacterial agents, they are the natural choice for ensuring that the home is kept as germ free as possible which is particularly important when infants and children are around.

Essential oils also have the added bonus of a pleasant fragrance. Essential oils may be added to hot water and detergent for wiping down work surfaces, floors and equipment and are an effective and natural method for ensuring hygiene within the home. Essential oils are particularly useful in the nursery for equipment and furniture, the kitchen and bathroom.

Insect repellent – Apply essential oils neat to hard, non polished surfaces, diffuse in a light ring or electric diffuser or add to a water spray and sprayed as required to repel insects. Useful to repel mosquitos and other pests.

Massage – Add essential oils to a carrier oil suitable for skin type and apply to the body with long upward strokes. Use the recommended dilution. Useful to treat specific skin conditions, relaxation and general well being.

Scenting linen – A few drops of the colourless or lighter essential oils may be added to the final rinsing water when laundering. Care must be taken to avoid staining and damage to delicate fabrics. Particularly effective for keeping baby linen and clothes fresh and fragrant.

Shower – For older children who like to shower, add drops of essential oil to a washcloth, sponge or loofah which has been thoroughly wetted. Apply to the skin rubbing briskly whilst remaining under the shower. Useful for general hygiene or to treat specific conditions.

Skin preparations – Essential oils may be added to creams and lotions for skin care and are particularly useful for application to prevent chaffing and nappy rash. Either add to bland, lanolin free commercial preparations or prepare your own base creams using natural ingredients. Refreshing skin toners or spritzers may be prepared by adding essential oils to spring water and applying to the skin with a spray. This is a useful method of refreshing and cooling the skin to soothe and calm. Bath and shower preparations may be formulated by adding the desired blend of essential oils to unfragranced foaming gels. Similarly, shampoo may be prepared by adding suitable essential oils to gentle shampoo bases. Useful for gentle cleansing of the skin and hair and to prevent dry scaly skin and scalp.

Steam inhalation – Essential oils may be added to a bowl of hot water and inhaled under a towel. Essential oils may also be added to a facial steamer. One drop of essential oil maximum. This is useful for those conditions listed above and also for congested skin conditions.

Vapourisation – Essential oils may be added to vapourising light rings, diffusers, electric vapourising stones or onto a cotton wool ball placed on a radiator to diffuse the fragrant molecules into the atmosphere which can affect the infant or child's physiological or psychological condition according to the properties of the oil or oils chosen. This is a simple and effective way to use essential oils for both treatment and environmental fragrancing. This is a useful method for use with colds, coughs, congestion, asthma and sinus problems.

13 | Conditions

The following is a list of conditions which may benefit from the use of essential oils and the suggested oils for their treatment. As you become familiar with essential oils and confident in their use you will find that you discover many properties for yourself.

Do remember, however, that the effects of essential oils may vary when used on certain conditions and that treatment may take longer than conventional methods.

Aching muscles – Tea Tree, Lavender.

Allergies – Lavender, Roman Chamomile.

Asthma – Roman Chamomile, Lavender.

Bites and stings – Tea Tree, Lavender.

Boils – Lavender, Tea Tree.

Bruises – Lavender, Tea Tree.

Burns – Lavender.

Catarrh – Lavender, Tea Tree, Eucalyptus.

Chillblains – Lavender, Rose.

Colds and Flu – Tea Tree, Eucalyptus, Peppermint.

Cold Sores – Tea Tree, Lavender.

Colic – Mandarin, Fennel, Peppermint.

Cuts and Abrasions – Lavender, Tea Tree.

Constipation – Mandarin.

Cradle Cap – Lavender.

Dandruff – Tea Tree, Rose.

Digestive – Fennel, Mandarin, Peppermint.

Earache – Lavender, Tea Tree.

Eczema – Roman Chamomile, Lavender, Rose.

Fatigue – Mandarin, Rose, Lavender.

Flatulence – Fennel, Mandarin.

Haircare – Roman Chamomile, Lavender, Rose.

Headaches – Lavender, Peppermint.

Hygiene – Tea Tree, Lavender, Eucalyptus.

Immune System – Tea Tree, Lavender.

Infection – Roman Chamomile, Lavender, Tea Tree.

Insomnia – Lavender, Neroli, Rose.

Mouth Ulcers – Tea Tree.

Nausea – Peppermint.

Psoriasis – Roman Chamomile, Lavender.

Rashes – Lavender.

Ringworm - Tea Tree.

Scars – Lavender, Neroli, Mandarin.

Sinusitis – Tea Tree, Eucalyptus, Peppermint.

Sore Throat – Tea Tree, Lavender.

Spots – Tea Tree, Lavender.

Stress – Mandarin, Neroli.

Sunburn – Lavender, Tea Tree.

Thrush – Tea Tree, Lavender.

Toothache – Roman Chamomile, Lavender, Tea Tree.

Verrucas – Tea Tree.

Warts – Tea Tree.

14 | Simple massage blends

You may wish to formulate your own special massage blends to suit the mood and condition of the infant or child. To get you started, I have created several blends that are pleasant to use and delicately fragrant. Remember that you must always keep to the blending proportions given and ensure that the essential oils are well blended. Where several oils are required, formulate a synergistic blend.

Add essential oil to a carrier oil to suit the skin and as a general rule 10mls of carrier is sufficient for an infant or small child but for larger bodies, you may have to increase the amount of carrier oil.

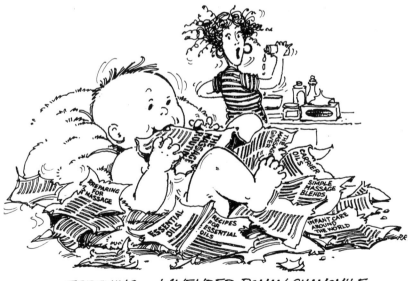

...TEETHING — LAVENDER, ROMAN CHAMOMILE...

Antiseptic – Lavender, Eucalyptus, Tea Tree.

Calming – Neroli.

Cold/Flu – Peppermint, Eucalyptus, Tea Tree.

Colic/Digestive – Fennel, Mandarin.

Dry skin – Lavender, Roman Chamomile.

Gentle – Rose.

Happy – Rose, Neroli.

Relaxation – Lavender.

Sensitive skin – Roman Chamomile.

Sleepy – Roman Chamomile, Lavender.

Soothing – Lavender, Mandarin.

Teething – Lavender, Roman Chamomile.

15 | Recipes for using essential oils

Aching Muscles – For general aches and to alleviate tension. Lavender and Tea Tree in a bath to soothe aches. Add 1 drop of each to a bath full of lukewarm water. Alternatively, add 1 drop of each oil to 10 mls of carrier oil.

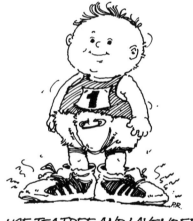

...USE TEA TREE AND LAVENDER...

Allergies – For minor allergies and to help strengthen the immune system to prevent further allergies occurring. Roman Chamomile in a diffuser is useful to help weaken allergies such as hay fever and pollen irritations. Add 1 drop to the diffuser. Lavender is soothing as a topical application in a cream or ointment base. Add 2 drops to 10 mls of base cream or carrier oil. Alternatively a Lavender bath is cooling and healing. Add 2 drops to a bath full of lukewarm water.

Asthma – To relax and calm spasmodic and irregular breathing, Roman Chamomile or Lavender gently allow breathing to return to normal. Add 1 drop for inhalation on a tissue or diffuser or massage the chest using 1 drop of oil to 10mls of carrier oil.

Bites and Stings – To soothe the discomfort and pain choose Tea Tree and Lavender. Wash the area with water to which a drop of either oil has been added. Remove the sting using sterile tweezers. Apply a cool compress to which Tea Tree has been added. Apply Lavender regularly until pain subsides.

Boils – To treat pain and infection use Lavender and Tea Tree. Make a compress using 1 drop of each oil in hot water and apply to the affected area.

Bruises – To alleviate pain and discolouration use Lavender and Tea Tree. Make a compress using 1 drop of each oil in cool water and apply to the affected area.

Burns – To heal and prevent scarring, Lavender applied neat to the injured area will soothe and relieve pain. Apply 1 drop of oil to the burn, and continue to apply at intervals until the area heals.

Catarrh – To relieve congestion and stuffiness use Lavender, Tea Tree and Eucalyptus. Mix 1 drop of each in an amber bottle. Add 1 drop to a diffuser. Also, add 1 drop to 10mls of carrier oil and massage the face, neck and chest. A drop of the blend applied to a pillow or tissue for an older child will also be helpful.

Chillblains – For painful and tender areas use Lavender or Rose. Add 1 drop of either oil to a footbath. Gently apply 1 drop Rose oil in 10mls of Evening Primrose oil. As a preventative measure massage the feet regularly with the above blend to stimulate healthy circulation.

Colds and Flu – To help with all the symptoms which cause discomfort use Tea Tree, Eucalyptus and Peppermint. Mix 1 drop of each in an amber bottle. Add 1 drop to a diffuser. Also add 2 drops to a lukewarm bath.

Cold Sore – To soothe pain and strengthen the immune system to help prevent further attacks use Tea Tree and Lavender. Mix 1 drop of each oil in an amber bottle. Add 1 drop to a cotton bud and apply neat to the affected area. Add 2 drops to a lukewarm bath. Use the blend in the bath regularly as a preventative measure.

Colic – To soothe discomfort use Mandarin and Fennel. Mix 1 drop of each in an amber bottle and add 1 drop to 10mls of carrier oil. Massage over the abdomen and chest in a clockwise direction. Add 1 drop of this blend to a lukewarm bath also to ease discomfort.

Constipation – To gently relieve discomfort use Mandarin. Add 1 drop to 10mls of carrier oil and massage the abdomen in a clockwise direction.

Cradle Cap – To soften the scalp, and allow this condition to be treated whilst also preventing re-occurrence use Lavender. Add 1 drop of Lavender to Jojoba and apply generously to the scalp. Allow the mixture to remain on the scalp for as long as possible before removing with a gentle shampoo base. Repeat the treatment regularly until condition is cleared and then as a preventative measure.

Cuts and Abrasions – For general antiseptic and healing properties use Lavender and Tea Tree. Wash the area with water to which a drop of either oil has been added. Apply Tea Tree neat to the area 3 times per day until healing is complete. Add these oils to a fragrance free cream base for use as an effective antiseptic cream. Add 2 drops of each oil to 10mls of cream base.

Dandruff – To gently detoxify a scaly dry scalp use Tea Tree and Rose. Mix 1 drop of each in an amber bottle. Add 1 drop to 10mls of Jojoba and apply generously to the scalp. Allow the mixture to remain on the scalp overnight if possible before removing with a gentle shampoo base. Use regularly until the condition clears.

Digestive Problems – For all digestive problems use Fennel, Mandarin and Peppermint. Mix 1 drop of each in an amber bottle. Add 1 drop to a diffuser. Also add 2 drops to a lukewarm bath or 1 drop to 10mls of carrier oil and massage the abdomen and chest.

Earache – To soothe pain and discomfort use Tea Tree, Lavender and Roman Chamomile. Mix 1 drop of each in an amber bottle. Make a compress using 1 drop in warm water. Also, add 1 drop to 10mls of carrier oil and gently apply behind the ears.

Eczema – For the relief of irritation use Roman Chamomile, Lavender or Rose. Add 1 drop of either of these oils to a lukewarm bath. Add 1 drop of Roman Chamomile to 25mls of Jojoba and Avocado oil and gently apply to affected areas.

Fatigue – To ease fatigue and promote well-being use Mandarin, Rose or Lavender. Add 1 drop of either of these oils to a lukewarm bath. Add 1 drop of oil and gently apply to affected areas.

Flatulence – To relieve discomfort and bloating use Fennel or Mandarin. Add 1 drop of each in an amber bottle and add 1 drop to 10mls of carrier oil. Massage over the abdomen in a clockwise direction. Add 1 drop to warm water and apply a compress to the abdomen. Repeat the procedure until the condition has eased.

Haircare – To promote healthy hair and scalp use Roman Chamomile, Lavender or Rose. Add 1 drop of either oil to 10mls Jojoba and apply to the scalp and hair massaging gently but firmly to stimulate circulation. Allow the oil to remain on the scalp and hair for as long as possible before removing with a gentle shampoo base. Repeat the treatment regularly to keep the scalp healthy and the hair in good condition.

Headaches – To relieve headaches use Lavender or Peppermint. Apply 1 drop of either oil to a diffuser or for inhalation on a tissue. Add 1 drop of Lavender to 10mls Jojoba and gently massage the temples in circular movement to ease tense muscles and relieve pain.

Hygiene – For general hygiene within the home choose Tea Tree, Lavender and Eucalyptus. Mix 10 drops of each oil in an amber bottle and add several drops to hot soapy water for cleaning work surfaces, floors in the home. This blend is particularly useful for bathroom, nursery or sick room. Use regularly as part of your cleaning regime.

Immune system – To strengthen and increase natural immunity use Tea Tree and Lavender. Mix 1 drop of each in an amber bottle and add 1 drop to a lukewarm bath. Add 1 drop to 10mls of Sweet Almond oil and massage the body. This treatment is useful to help prevent colds and simple ailments.

Infection – To help fight infection and promote healing use Roman Chamomile, Lavender and Tea Tree. Mix 1 drop of each in an amber bottle and add 1 drop to a lukewarm bath. Massage is not advisable if infection is present but a compress with 1 drop of the blend is helpful applied to the affected area.

Insomnia – To aid restful sleep choose from Lavender, Neroli or Rose. Add 1 drop of either oil to a lukewarm bath and follow this with a soothing massage using 1 drop of the same essential oil to 10mls of Sweet Almond oil each evening before bed.

Mouth Ulcers – To ease stinging and pain whilst promoting healing, use Tea Tree. Add 1 drop of Tea Tree to 10mls of warm water, agitate vigorously to disperse the essential oil and apply to the affected area with a cotton bud. Apply regularly to the affected areas. Older children could gargle with the mixture, but care must be taken not to swallow any of the liquid.

Nausea – To bring relief use Peppermint. Add 1 drop to a diffuser or 1 drop applied to a tissue. Use when travelling as a preventative measure and whenever the atmosphere is stuffy.

Psoriasis – To soothe, heal and prevent discomfort use Roman Chamomile and Lavender. Mix 1 drop of each in an amber bottle. Add 1 drop to a lukewarm bath. Add 1 drop to 10mls of base oil and gently smooth over affected areas. Apply several times daily. In extreme cases add 1 drop to 10mls of Jojoba and apply liberally over affected areas. Repeat the treatment until the skin returns to normal and use the blend regularly to ensure that the condition is kept under control.

Rashes – To soothe discomfort and itchy, irritated skin use Lavender. Bathe the area with water to which 1 drop of

Lavender has been added. Lavender is soothing as a topical application in a cream or ointment base. Add 2 drops to 10mls of base cream. Apply to the affected area until discomfort subsides.

Ringworm – To fight fungal infection and ease discomfort use Tea Tree. Add 1 drop to a lukewarm bath. Add Tea Tree neat to affected area 3 times per day. Ensure that towels, linen etc are kept exclusively for the affected child as this condition may be spread through contract with contaminated items.

Scars – To heal scar tissue and refine skin texture use Lavender, Mandarin or Neroli. Apply Lavender neat to the area to speed the healing process, repeat 3 times daily. When healing has taken place massage the area daily with 1 drop of either oil in 10mls of Evening Primrose oil or Wheatgerm oil. Use firm frictions over the scar tissue to ensure that healing takes place in a uniform manner. Continue this treatment until redness and scarring have diminished.

Sinusitis – To ease congestion and prevent sinus infection use Tea Tree, Eucalyptus and Peppermint. Mix 1 drop of each in an amber bottle and add 1 drop to a diffuser. Massage the face, concentrating on the forehead, nose and cheek areas with 1 drop of oil to 10mls of carrier oil. a warm compress using the same blend may also bring relief when applied to the facial area.

Sore throat – To alleviate discomfort use Tea Tree and Lavender. Mix 1 drop of each in an amber bottle and make up a warm compress using 1 drop and apply to the throat area. Add 1 drop of oil to 10mls carrier oil and apply liberally to the throat and jaw area. Older children could gargle with 1 drop to 10mls of warm water but care must be taken not to swallow any of the liquid.

Spots – To fight infection and heal use Tea Tree and Lavender. Mix 1 drop of each in an amber bottle. Apply the neat with a cotton bud directly to the spot avoiding surrounding skin. Repeat 3 times daily.

Sunburn – To cool and soothe the skin use Tea Tree and Lavender. Mix 1 drop of each in an amber bottle. Add 2 drops to a cool bathe and immerse the body completely. Add 1 drop to 25mls Natural Yogurt and apply liberally to the affected areas.

Stress – To relax, calm and restore well-being use Mandarin or Neroli. Add 1 drop of either oil to a warm bath. Add 1 drop of essential oil to 10mls carrier oil and massage the body. Repeat this treatment regularly to ensure that stress levels are reduced.

Toothache – To ease pain and discomfort of toothache or teething use Roman Chamomile, Lavender and Tea Tree. Mix 1 drop of each in an amber bottle. Make a warm compress using 1 drop of the mix. Apply regularly to the affected side.

Thrush – To fight this condition use Tea Tree and Lavender. Mix 1 drop of each in an amber bottle. Add 2 drops to a warm bath. Add 1 drop to 10mls Soya Bean oil and massage the body. Repeat this treatment morning and evening to ensure that the condition clears.

Veruccas – To fight this condition use Tea Tree. Apply neat to the affected area using a cotton bud. Cover the area with a sterile dressing and repeat the application 3 times daily. Ensure that the affected area is kept covered as this infection may spread. To strengthen the immune system add 2 drops of Tea Tree to the daily bath.

Warts – To remove unsightly growths use Tea Tee. Apply neat to the affected area with a cotton bud. Cover the area with a sterile dressing and repeat the application 3 times daily. To strengthen the immune system and 2 drops of Tea Tree to the daily bath.

16 | Conclusion

Now that you have tried these simple massage techniques and sampled the delightful aromas of essential oils and aroma-therapy, I am sure that you will be keen to include them in your daily baby and childcare routine. I hope that you enjoy using this book and that you and your baby spend many happy times together!

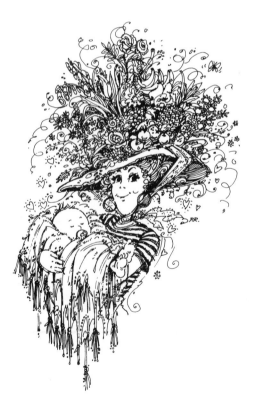

OTHER BOOKS FROM AMBERWOOD PUBLISHING ARE:

Aromatherapy Lexicon – The Essential Reference by Geoff Lyth and Sue Charles is a colourful, fun way to learn about Aromatherapy. £4.99.

Aromatherapy – A Guide for Home Use by Christine Westwood. All you need to know about essential oils and using them. £1.99.

Aromatherapy – For Stress Management by Christine Westwood. Covering the use of essential oils for everyday stress-related problems. £2.99.

Aromatherapy – For Healthy Legs and Feet by Christine Westwood. A guide to the use of essential oils for the treatment of legs and feet. £2.99.

Aromatherapy – Simply For You by Marion Del Gaudio Mak. A clear, simple and comprehensive guide to Aromatherapy for beginners. £1.99.

Aromatherapy – A Nurses Guide by Ann Percival SRN. The ultimate, safe, lay guide to the natural benefits of Aromatherapy. Including recipes and massage techniques for many medical conditions and a quick reference chart. £2.99.

Aromatherapy – A Nurses Guide for Women by Ann Percival SRN. Concentrates on women's health for all ages. Including sections on PMT, menopause, infertility, cellulite. £2.99.

Aromatherapy – Essential Oils in Colour by Rosemary Caddy Bsc Hons, ARCS MISP is a unique book depicting the chemistry of Essential oils. £9.99.

Aroma Science – The Chemistry & Bioactivity of Essential Oils by Dr Maria Lis-Balchin. With a comprehensive list of the Oils and scientific analysis. Includes sections on the sense of smell and the history of Aromatherapy. £4.99.

Plant Medicine – A Guide for Home Use (New Edition) by Charlotte Mitchell MNIMH. A guide to home use giving an insight into the wonderful healing qualities of plants. £2.99.

Woman Medicine – Vitex Agnus Castus by Simon Mills MA, FNIMH. The story of the herb that has been used for centuries in the treatment of women's problems. £2.99.

Ancient Medicine – Ginkgo Biloba (New Edition) by Dr Desmond Corrigan BSc(Pharms), MA, Phd, FLS, FPSI. Improved memory, circulation and concentration are associated with Ginkgo and explained in this book. £2.99.

Indian Medicine – The Immune System by Dr Desmond Corrigan BSc(Pharms), MA, Phd, FLS, FPSI. An intriguing account of the history of the plant called Echinacea and its power to influence the immune system. £2.99.

Herbal Medicine for Sleep & Relaxation by Dr Desmond Corrigan BSc(Pharms), MA, PhD, FLS, FPSI. A guide to the natural sedatives as an alternative to orthodox drug therapies, drawing on the latest medical research, presented in an easy reference format. £2.99.

Herbal First Aid by Andrew Chevallier BA, MNIMH. A beautifully clear reference book of natural remedies and general first aid in the home. £2.99.

Natural Taste – Herbal Teas, A Guide for Home Use by Andrew Chevallier BA, MNIMH. Contains a comprehensive compendium of Herbal Teas gives information on how to make it, its benefits, history and folklore. £2.99.

Garlic– How Garlic Protects Your Heart by Prof E. Ernst MD, PhD. Used as a medicine for over 4500 years, this book examines the latest scientific evidence supporting Garlic's effect in reducing cardiovascular disease, the Western World's number one killer. £3.99.

Insomnia – Doctor I Can't Sleep by Dr Adrian Williams FRCP. Written by one of the world's leading sleep experts, Dr Williams explains the phenomenon of sleep and sleeping disorders and gives advice on treatment. With 25% of the adult population reporting difficulties sleeping – this book will be essential reading for many. £2.99.

Signs & Symptoms of Vitamin Deficiency by Dr Leonard Mervyn BSc, PhD, C.Chem, FRCS. A home guide for self diagnosis which explains and assesses Vitamin Therapy for the prevention of a wide variety of diseases and illnesses. £2.99.

Causes & Prevention of Vitamin Deficiency by Dr Leonard Mervyn BSc, PhD, C.Chem, FRCS. A home guide to the Vitamin content of foods and the depletion caused by cooking, storage and processing. It includes advice for those whose needs are increased due to lifestyle, illness etc. £2.99.

Eyecare Eyewear – For Better Vision by Mark Rossi Bsc, MBCO. A complete guide to eyecare and eyewear including an assessment of the types of spectacles and contact lenses available and the latest corrective surgical procedures. £3.99.

Arthritis and Rheumatism by Dr John Cosh FRCP, MD. Covers all forms of Arthritis, its affects and the treatments available. £4.95.